Practical Asperger Syndrome Manual

Dawn Lucan

This book is a culmination of my own thoughts and personal experiences regarding my own diagnosis of Asperger Syndrome. The opinions stated in this book are of the author. This book is no substitute for professional advice in the fields of education, legal, medical, or therapeutic.

Practical Asperger Syndrome Manual

Copyright © 2010 by Dawn Lucan

Library of Congress Cataloging –in- Publication Data

Lucan, Dawn

Practical Asperger Syndrome Manual

ISBN 978-0-557-72875-6

1. Asperger Syndrome 2. Asperger Syndrome Parenting 3. Asperger Syndrome Education 4. Asperger Syndrome Diet

To my brother, you inspire me every day.

To my mother, thank you for helping me become who I am.

To my friends, you inspire me every day.

Foreword

I began writing Practical Asperger Syndrome to help parents understand this complex disability. As a person diagnosed with Asperger Syndrome, I have faced many interesting challenges over time. Each challenge made me stronger in life. I know others need help getting stronger to help their disabled child or teen grow stronger in life.

I began my life journey towards writing this book more than a decade ago. I taught two enrichment courses over the web focusing on parents and educators. Though the courses, I hoped to create teamwork and better understanding of disabled students in the classroom.

I used a combination of book knowledge and personal experience to help both parents and educators. Over a period of three years, I reached more than an estimated thousand parents and educators. I know through my work that more lives were touched by those courses than those who registered, took, and read the course material.

As time progressed, I became interested in writing various books to help parents. I wanted to reach parents who might not surf the web on a regular basis.

I noticed how parents wanted information on how they could help their disabled child succeed in life. They also wanted ways to parent and help their child. The reason was that there were few books out there on parenting a disabled child.

I really enjoyed writing this book. I hope you get as much pleasure from reading it as I had writing it for you. I really enjoy sharing my personal and educational experiences with other people. I know there is much to learn by them. I also know your child or teen diagnosed with Asperger Syndrome will benefit from this book.

Dawn Lucan

Table of Contents

Introduction

For as long as I can remember, I have been different. I did not know how or why. I just knew that I behaved and sounded different than the other neighborhood kids. Later, it included my classmates in school.

It was not until my Father's fiancé later third wife encouraged me to search for answers. I was diagnosed for the longest time with Attention Deficit Hyperactive Disorder with the inattentive form. It was a diagnosis given to me during my preteen years. I also had the diagnosis of being learning disabled.

I was young when a neighbor noticed that I was developing differently from the other children. This happened during the early 1970s. I started receiving help from professionals from then on with the characteristics of my unknown disability.

I had received help during my school years in the form of Special Education. I had attended small classes from the time I entered first grade. I graduated from high school receiving help in the resource classroom room setting.

I did great academically. I did not struggle in the resource room as much. I did struggle some with the mainstream classroom. It was entirely not academic in nature. I had a number of struggles with my fine motor skills. I could not handle intensive writing classes well. I got overwhelmed at times with it.

I had a major difficulty with individuals teasing me almost throughout my school years. There were a couple of years when I was not teased by someone. My bullies primarily focused on my appearance which meant body and clothing.

I had trouble finding a group of friends to associate with during school hours. Most individuals ignored me. I did find a helpful group of friends during my senior year of high school when I joined a school band as a manager.

I dreamed of being a teacher from a young age. I played with my few friends about being a teacher. I always thought it was possible.

I did attend college as an education major. I did great academic wise. I still had some problems social wise. I did not know how to fit in with any campus crowd just like I did during my school years. I did participate with some clubs though. I did not graduate with teacher certification.

I did work after graduation. It took a bit of work since I did not interview well in person. I could read very little body language.

There were two attempts at getting me help during my childhood. I did have a little success with the psychological therapy during my childhood. I did receive a diagnosis of Attention Deficit Hyperactive Disorder. The diagnosis was later discarded in 1996 when I was diagnosed with a form of Mild Autism.

After moving to Michigan in 1996, I became interested in finding a diagnosis that fit me. It came after being encouraged by my future step mother to search for one. She worked as a social worker who worked at an adult day care.

I first tried a psychiatrist for a diagnosis. I spent a number of weeks seeing him. It was covered by my insurance. He gave me medication for anxiety. However, he did not find a cause for my anxiety.

After a while, my father and future step mother decided to try a second place. It was a nonprofit which serviced both Autistic and developmentally disabled adults.

We believed it would work in finding a diagnosis. We thought they knew all levels of Autism since they worked with lower functioning adults. The place seemed to be perfect fit in finding the services needed to help me at the time.

The intake worker was fantastic. He seemed to notice my difficulties very well. The evaluation went well. However, it was difficult getting the results. The person had a difficult time believing I was on the Autism spectrum. The results were disheartening.

I decided to research before trying to get an evaluation. I heard that a major state university had an Autism Department. I decided to try there. I had no luck in finding it. I tried the university's telephone system and the university's website.

I decided to try the Autism Society located within the state for my next attempt. I talked to someone over the telephone, and I was referred to two different doctors in my county.

After talking to both places, I decided to go with one place. My health insurance was not taken there. It did not bother me at all. I just wanted an accurate diagnosis. I had to wait several months before I could be seen. It worked! I was accurately diagnosed with Mild Autism for the first time in my entire life.

I felt relieved once I had my diagnosis. I finally had the answers that I had been searching for consciously or unconsciously for years. It was all thanks to a family member who encouraged me to search for answers. I felt like I had some closure in my life when it came to finding answers.

About Your Child

You have spent many sleepless nights trying to discover what is wrong or different about your child. You have finally got the diagnosis. Where do you go from here after receiving it?

The biggest thing to remember is that your child has not changed at all. The only thing that has changed is that there is a name to your child's problems that he or she is facing on a regular basis. The other thing is that you are not alone in facing these problems.

Remember your child still has the same gifts given to him or her before she received the diagnosis. They have a talent in something which will develop in time just like any other child.

Your child will always have some sort of interest. It sort of takes the form of a fixation of interest. They will want to learn everything they can about it. At times, they will even want to observe it in more detail. This parenting and personality trait can work to your advantage at times with things.

Consistency will benefit your child in more ways than one. Many on the Autism spectrum including Mild Autism prefer having consistency in their lives. It could be a predictable schedule or even a checklist. Having a large task broken down into its smaller parts can help your child, too.

You can utilize it as enrichment material with learning a new educational concept. For example, you can turn it into solving word problems if they are struggling to learn it. It will make the child want to learn even more about it.

Your child loves to research about their current fixation in many different ways. It can be used as an advantage to get them to read more about it. The library becomes your ally in finding books about it.

I recommend taking a deep breath because things can improve with the right help. He or she may not always be the perfect child every moment of the day. However, his or her coping mechanisms for dealing with their disability can improve.

Your significant other or spouse can help or hinder your child in developing. The trick is to learn their unique abilities in order to help you in ways that are beneficial to help your disabled child.

Your spouse or significant other may or may not accept the diagnosis right away if ever. His or her response to the diagnosis may take one of several different forms.

They may want to place the blame on you for something out of your control. Remind them that blaming someone for genetics does not help the child. You can try to encourage them to help with things to encourage personal growth in the child. Show your spouse or significant other how they can help you with them. It may take time before this happens.

The hardest one to deal with is the denial of the problem. It could stem from one of several different reasons. One reason could be that they could have it undiagnosed. A different reason could be that they believe the child is acting just like a normal child.

Find little things for them to help with on a regular basis to help you. Do it without nagging about it. It does not have to be child related. It could be helping around the house. Share the impact which it could have for him or her in the future if done. For example, it could be more energy for watching a favorite television show you both enjoy watching together.

Your spouse or significant other might have the diagnosis in himself or herself. It could be diagnosed or undiagnosed. If undiagnosed, the problem could have been ignored for years. This denial can have a huge impact on their parenting of the child.

If the parent is showing signs of Mild Autism, there is help for you. Their denials can take a couple of forms. However, you can also use their best qualities to help you help your Autistic child.

Utilize their strengths in assisting you. For example, if they are good at computers, they can share what they have learned over time. Their fixations on a subject can be a huge asset at times when researching a particular subject to help your disabled child.

Encourage him or her to find help some form of help. They can become a role model for the child in seeking help.

Encourage role modeling behavior. Have them show positive attributes in front of the child. Those individuals with Mild Autism learn by mimicking sometimes. You can give them some signal when they are doing great or correct when necessary on their behavior.

The second type is avoidance and the belief it is just a developmental stage that will vanish with maturity. It is a hard sell. The person might believe it based on the assumption every child is like it at one point or another in his or her lifetime.

Someone could be pressuring them on the child being normal. It could be a family member, medical professional, or even a teacher. The person could believe give it a little time, and the child will grow in maturity. You are arguing against two or more people in this case.

Avoidance could create problems with consistency with therapeutic and parenting methods. The reason is there is no agreement with the parenting method between the parents. It could create confusion for the child in regards to the schedule or expectations.

Avoidance approach can sometimes create worse behavior problems in your child. The mixed signals could create confusion with the child on their expectations. As a result, they do not learn the proper social and behavioral expectations for a social situation or interaction.

The third type is the fix it mode. They are trying to find a quick fix to help your child overcome his or her disability. He or she might research possible cures on the web or read books on it. These approaches may or may not work.

You can actually work with this kind of acceptance in a team parenting approach. However, there might be a problem or two which might occur from time to time due to a lack of communication between the two of you on things.

You can utilize him or her to research the latest parenting or educational methods. There are new books, magazines, and websites which come out on a regular basis on a variety of topics. The key is to get them to share their findings with you before implementing them. Otherwise, you could find them undermining your decisions regarding your child.

The trick is to remind them to be patient during the process because any new method needs time to work. It does not matter if it is a new parenting method or therapy. It takes time and patience to implement and work effectively.

In addition, you need to remind them about it being a team effort. If you two do not work as a team, the new method will not work. Neither one should undermine the other.

Undermining your partner and team member can take the form of correcting them in front of the child. Your corrections should be done in private. Consistency is the key to the new method taking hold and working with your child when it comes to new utilizing new parenting methods.

If a new treatment method is located, you need to consult or need to encourage approaching the doctor or therapist. They know if the treatment will work against any current medical treatment. There is a computer system which will help him judge if it will be harmful to your child.

Acceptance is the final parenting mode. They work with you on parenting and punishment mode. They provide assistance in whichever way that helps you such as handling appointments. They make it a true team effort for the benefit of the child.

Is there any common advice to follow in making my quality of life easier with this disability? Yes, there are things you can do to improve your quality of life.

Suggest tasks to them to help you with taking care of the child. Do not use a nag and instead use a helpful tone. Show appreciation for their help before, during and after the task. This will encourage them to help more often.

There are things you can do no matter how cooperative the other parent is with you. It can help ease the parenting tension.

Take time for yourselves no matter what. Raising a disabled child is a difficult task. It could be individual or couples time. It gives you a chance to recharge your mental batteries.

Gently remind yourself there will always be a difference of opinions on things. Even among parents have the same belief and parenting system, there will always be differences. The trick is how both of you handle the difference of opinions on things.

Join a support group. The local hospital or school social worker will have a list of them. They are great when you are facing a problem related to the disability. In addition, there are people with varying degrees of experience with it.

Keep a diary of things related to his disability. It could be of medical, personal, and educational stuff. You have no idea when it would come in handy in the future.

Never stop learning or researching about the disability. There is always new research material coming out. Some of it could help you with raising your child. The local intermediate unit or college library would have access to these research journals. In addition, some of these journals can be located on the web for free.

Put time aside each day to communicate with each other. Select a time of day that works for both of you. It could be about any issue or even your day. It could be as little as sharing accomplishments or problems. The main thing is not to be judgmental. Communication is important no matter what to making a relationship work.

Remember to give verbal or written praise for their accomplishments no matter how big or small. Positive feedback can make a great impact on him or her on how they view and handle things.

If you have a normal developing child, make time for him or her on a regular basis. When you have a disabled child, it is really easy to focus more on the disabled child.

There is no single approach in handling a child with Asperger Syndrome. The main thing is to remember is that your child is more than their disability. You are not helpless in helping them become a productive adult. It does not have to cost any money.

In later chapters, you will learn some skills that I found important in helping your child at home, school, and in your local community.

Dietary Ideas

As I began writing this book, I began to think about what ideas I could to help a parent with their disabled child's diet. I know most parents worry about the cost involved with their budget. As a disabled person, I watch my budget carefully. I am no different with the grocery store. There are simple things you can do to help your child and enhance their diet.

Create homemade juice popsicles. All you would need to do is buy the fruit juice at your local grocery store and pour it into a mold. There are reusable molds out on the market. You can use your child's favorite fruit juices.

Use a juicer and create your own natural juices. You can buy fresh fruits and vegetables at the local grocery store.

Substitute spaghetti sauce for ketchup with recipes. It can add both flavor and nutrition into the recipe and your child's diet.

Add a nutritional supplement into your pudding recipes or boxed puddings. Many come in powdered form besides the liquid form.

Add a nutritional supplement powder into your child's milk. There are some fantastic flavors out there. Some are pretty affordable.

Add milk to your child's hot chocolate.

Add a chocolate nutritional supplement powder to your child's milk to make chocolate milk.

Add a nutritional supplement to your child's milkshake. There are good tasting and affordable ones on the market.

Add applesauce into your baking. Many cake boxes have applesauce as an alternative to oil or butter into the mix. It is very easy to do.

Add pureed vegetables into various side dishes. I recommend using the same colored vegetable, so it would not give it away as being different from the normal kind. For example, corn would be a fantastic mix in for macaroni and cheese.

Use cornmeal or rice instead of bread crumbs in your recipes.

Make your stuffing with rice instead of bread crumbs.

Create fruit smoothies in your blender using juice and a fruit or two for your child.

Make pies using a crushed cereal pie crust. The crust is both colorful and nutritious.

It does not have to cost a lot to feed your disabled child healthy foods. With a few simple ingredients added into your recipes, you can add nutrition into your child's diet.

Sensory Issues

Children with Autism can have sensory issues and how they process it through their brains. It can create a variety of different issues with their daily life. How does it impact them? What can be done to help him or her with their sensory issues?

What are the five senses? They are sight, hearing, touch, and smell. It is through the senses how your child perceives the world around them each day.

Information is processed through their sense like their fingers touching the surface of an object. The information is then moved through your child's nerves to the brain. Their brain then processes and then interprets the sensory information given to it by your child's finger tips.

An Autistic child has problems processing the sensory information given to them by their brain. This will sometime create problems for them.

The sensory integration problem can show in a variety of different methods. I know when I am having sensory integration problems by having a headache. The headache will often vanish after I leave the situation.

How can you help your Autistic child with their sensory issues? Are there any strategies or coping mechanisms that they can learn in how to deal with their sensory integration issues?

At school, you can request an Occupational Therapy evaluation. They will evaluate your child's needs regarding their small motor skills. During each session, the therapist will utilize exercises to improve their small motor skills.

Second, have a space set aside where your child could go when they have sensory issues at school. This item would need to be written into your child's I.E.P. This should not be used in a penalty situation for your child.

Third, check into your child receiving Sensory Integration Therapy at school. The sessions are done by an occupational therapist. It may or may not happen. During the therapy sessions, they will utilize therapeutic exercise methods to help calm and integrate your child's senses with their environment.

Fourth, check into your child receiving Sensory Integration Therapy at school. It may or may not happen. During the therapy sessions, they will use a therapeutic exercise method to help your child integrate their senses.

Fifth, avoid crowd situations if you can at times. If it gets too loud, your child will many times attempt to escape you. It will make it harder for you to locate them.

Finally, learn to brush your child's back. It is a calming method to their senses. It will help ease their senses back to normal when they are having problems with them.

Asperger Syndrome children and teens are known to have sensory integration problems. This problem will happen in a variety of different situations. If you use the right preventive methods, your child will learn how to deal with their sensory overload situations.

Friendship and Social Issues

Friendships are one of the hardest things to deal with Asperger Syndrome child. It is because you see your child wanting to have friends but struggles to have a single friend. You begin to wonder how to help them locate a friend. I will cover some of the problems and solutions to help them create a healthy relationship.

The hardest thing to watch is your child attempt to become friends with someone. It is not an easy process for them. The friendship process can lead to some problems every time that they attempt to make a new friend.

The copying behavior can be good or bad depending on it. It could range from cursing to imitating an action. The trick is to notice a new pattern early before it takes hold. Otherwise, it could take a while to get it out of their system.

How can you notice when a new friendship attempt is happening? You will begin to hear about a new friend or an attempt at one. It will be a bit obsessive at first with how they approach it during a conversation. Does the person acknowledge or notice your child? I am unable to describe it further because each child is different in their approach.

If the other child responds negatively or ignores your child, your child might try harder to become his or her friend.

Can you turn this into a lesson for your son or daughter? Yes, you can. You can turn it into a social story or practice with them on how to become a friend.

Before you can start the process of helping fix it, you need to find out what is going wrong. You can have a pretend session. It could be hard depending on how well your child does pretend play with other children.

It may take a bit of time getting out of the parent and child interaction. It depends on how well your child does pretend play or imagination. If they have trouble with it, it could take a couple of different approaches before it works. While doing it, pay attention to the body language and word usage during the conversation. It will tell you a lot about the situation at hand.

Also, watch how they interact at the next club meeting, sports meeting, or in public. Let them know in advance you are just monitoring things to help them out. It can tell you much about how they interact with their normal developing aged peers.

As you pay attention, there are important points to ponder about how your child holds a conversation. It is more than the length and how it starts off. There are several things you should look for during this time.

Observe how your child reacts to eye contact from the other child. Does your child go along with it or does your child react?

Observe how your child reacts to the other child's questions. Does he or she focus on their interests only and not the question? Do they answer the question with just a yes or no matter what is asked by the other child or person?

Observe how they handle conversations? Is it a two way conversation? How long does the conversation last? Is there a focus on their interests only? Is there any interest in the other child's interests? Does your child try to divert the conversation only to their interests?

Observe how they greet the other child. Does your child greet by name if they know it? How fast does he or she react back when greeted by another person?

Observe how your child does around visitors at home. Does he or she greet them? Does your child take an interest in them? Does your child try to initiate or engage them in a conversation? Does your child ignore the visitor?

After you have done all your observations, you need to come up with a game plan to help your child. You need to outline the concepts that your child needs to learn and the steps to accomplish them. The steps need to be broken down into smaller more understandable steps.

When you approach your child about it, you might want to give it a positive title which describes it well. For example, you might want to name it Project Friendship or some other catchy name.

Remind your child that it is not a quick process to learn this. Praise every small accomplishment or step mastered. Remind him or her that she did not master some new skills in a day in the past. Remind them to have patience because it is a work in progress to learn how to become a good friend.

At home, you can create play groups for disabled children. You can often find other parents interested in one at support groups, schools, or organizations. In these situations, you will find other parents interested in starting and belonging to a play group for disabled kids.

You should teach your child the signs of a good and bad friendship. It may take a lot of practice and review to teach them this skill. You can do this when you review how their day went at school. It can be a quick and easy conversation to have at times. It will take time and practice on your part to get the right information out of your child. Besides, it will benefit them well into adulthood.

There are things you set up at school to help your child learn social skills and building friendships. You will need to work with the school's staff and teachers to make it happen.

The first is request social skills therapy. To accomplish this, you will need an Individual Education Plan (also known as an I.E.P.). It is when the school's speech therapist will work with your child in an individual or group setting to learn the basics of social skills.

You can also suggest a circle of friends be done at school. It is when the teacher assigns selected small group students to be buddies with your disabled child. The entire situation is done in a controlled manner. Then, the teacher provides opportunities at school for your child to interact with them.

In the end, it will be well worth it once your child masters this new skill. Once your child starts developing new friendships, it will be well worth the time and effort it took to bring it about.

The Bullying Issue

Teasing, taunting and more can happen at school for your child. The problem dates back to further back than when you were a child or teenager. How do you handle this issue as a parent when it happens to your child or teen diagnosed with Asperger Syndrome?

The main problem with bullying is that a child or teen selects their victim their on looks or behavior. Some of these things can be changed, and other things cannot be changed easy. The thing is to change your child's or teen's response to it. The bully wants a negative reaction from them.

Your child's or teen's response can vary depending on their basic understanding of social situations. They can basically ignore it and then tell you about it. Some may think it was an attempt at them wanting to be a friend.

Should you intervene with the principal on your child's or teen's behalf at school? You should if the situation is ignored by the teacher or principal. In addition, the situation should not be ignored if your child or teen is being threatened with physical harm by another student.

There are laws out there against bullying another student at school. The law is there to protect your child or teen along with anyone else who is being bullied at school. It is your school's job to handle these school bullying incidents in a fair and effective manner.

You need to push for the school to start a bully prevention and peer mediation program at your school. The mediators are trained individuals who there to settle disputes between their peers. The person would step in when possibly a playground aide or teacher might not witness a situation. It can sometimes help a situation from becoming a larger and more difficult problem to deal with it.

As a parent, you should teach your child or teen to speak up against bullying against him or herself along with others. They should reach out to a teacher or principal when it happens. They should be reminded that the bullying will not stop until a responsible adult intervenes in the situation.

Bullying is a situation your Asperger Syndrome child or teen will most likely face at least once during their school career. With the right training and intervention, it can be handled right by you, your child, and the school staff.

Importance of Routines

Routines are very important to your child. It gives them a sense of consistency and predictability in their lives. Unpredictability can create problems for them at times. How can we help them?

A routine is a set of steps that a person follows to complete a task. In the chapter on lists, we covered the basic fundamentals of creating a basic checklist for your child or teen.

A problem with your child's routine can create problems for them. It can cause your child to act out or have behavior problems. In some cases, it can cause your child to have a meltdown or out of control behavior. These meltdowns can happen anywhere such as home, school, store, church, local park, etc.

For a child with Asperger Syndrome, a routine can bring normalcy to their world. Their world is full of distractions at times. The distractions can cause problems for them. It can also be a calming factor at times.

The first thing is to utilize checklists for important areas. It helps establish routines for the child. It gives them a list of expectations for a given task or a situation.

You can create a routine for almost anything that can happen during their daily life. For example, you can create one for chores, daily living skills, getting ready for school, etc.

Second, establish a daily schedule. It consists of the tasks or activities your child will do throughout their day. It gives them an idea of what to expect and when to expect it. You can adjust it as necessary.

The schedule can take a written form or a picture form. There is no exact single form it can take since it is dependent upon your child and their abilities.

It is also important to establish a routine at school for your child. It involves both you and your child's teacher working together as a team. There are things you can do to establish a routine.

First, you need to establish a daily communication journal between yourself and the teacher. You should update the teacher on important things related to the disability. The teacher should update you on how things are at school and any upcoming changes.

Second, have the teacher warn you when they or the shadow aid is not at school. This will help prevent any surprises or problems for the substitute teacher or paraprofessional.

Finally, have the school notify you if there are any changes in the schedule. It could be as small as a fire drill, class field trip, or school assembly. These could create behavior or adjustment problems in your child.

Routines are an important part of your Asperger Syndrome child's life. Simple daily routines designed specifically to the needs of your disabled child can make it easier for the both of you at the same time.

Life Skills Building

Just as you have utilized a checklist for certain daily life activities, a checklist can benefit your child, too. It has helped you organize your life better in areas such as grocery shopping. The same skill can bring better organization and expectations for your child.

A checklist helps in learning certain key every day concepts with your child. It can also be a reminder of what tasks need to be completed to do a basic chore or homework assignment. It can also bring predictability to your child.

If you notice, most everything you do in life is made up of lists. It is a basic concept of self organizing. By breaking up tasks for your child, you can teach them self organization skills as they grow older.

For a younger child unable to read, you might want to do a picture checklist. It is a group of pictures placed onto a cardboard or piece of paper in the order of completing the task.

For an older child such as a teen, you might want to work together to create and organize tasks into lists. This skill will help them build a skill necessary to enter the workforce. There is no exact age to start this stage. It is dependent upon your child's age and maturity.

It could be utilized to learn daily living skills such as hygiene or getting ready in the morning. As time your child becomes older, it becomes more automatic, and they will do it without a single reminder on your part.

It can take the form a basic checklist list of things needing to be completed. You can call it the morning ritual and night time ritual. It can include basic skills without going into detail once your child has mastered them.

For example for the morning ritual for a child before he or she reaches puberty age:

1. Get dressed into your clothing.
2. Brush your teeth.
3. Wash your face.
4. Comb or brush your hair.

At times, you might have a child who needs a more detailed list in order to have a task completed. The detailed list breaks down the task into greater detail than the basic checklist.

A checklist could be utilized for learning to clean a room. It could start off really basic with one task and then expanding it when your child masters it. A good place to start is with a basic organizing task.

For example a more detailed list might look like for a young child or someone who might need more detailed directions:

1. Pick up a toy.
2. Walk over to the toy chest.
3. Lift up the toy chest lid.
4. Place toy into the toy chest.
5. Start over at the number one task until all your toys are picked up.

The checklist can work with long complex long term homework assignments which might seem overwhelming. If the teacher does not break it up into smaller tasks, you can turn the larger assignment into smaller assignments yourself in the form of a checklist.

You can encourage your child to turn their homework assignments into a checklist. On a sheet of paper or daily planner, they would list their assignments. It would make it easier to track throughout the process.

Life skills building can take many different forms. I have only highlighted a couple of areas in which you could help your child. You could make a list for any task your child needs to accomplish on a daily or weekly basis. Just remember to break up the task into its simplest components.

Have some patience once you implement a checklist. It will take time for your child to adjust to it. With any new program you implement with your child, it takes time to adjust.

Activities, Clubs, and Sports

Asperger Syndrome children and teens are so capable despite being developmentally disabled. They might learn slower than the average person. Their disability does not get in the way of learning something new in life. They seek new learning opportunities just as we do in life.

Signing up your child for an activity is a great way to provide both learning new activities and meeting new friends. It also gives them new an opportunity at exploration.

As a parent, you have choices when it comes to selecting activities and clubs for your child. You could sign your child up for an inclusive setting or a disabled setting.

For sports, there are sports leagues designed for disabled children. You can find them through Special Olympics, Little League baseball, and even local YMCA. The registration fees may vary from organization to organization. Some organizations may offer free or low cost enrollment depending on your income and family size situation.

I know some organizations will want some parent involvement by you. Do not look at it as a bad experience or organization. Instead, look at it as individualized help for your child. Not every coach or scout leader knows how to work with the disabled.

Library events can provide a wonderful opportunity for your child to learn while attending a story hour. They can be introduced to the wonderful world of books through the love of a librarian. The activity is free to attend, but you will have to register your child in advance.

If you want to sign up your child for religious training, it is fine. Most churches or Sunday schools will work with you to help your child. They are firm believers in ministering to any individual from any background. They follow their religious instinct to share the word with anyone who wants to come and learn something new about their religion.

Any child loves learning new activities and participating in their local community. You can find activities at any price range to help your child grow into an adult. The organization might want your involvement on some level, but it is well worth it for your child's participation in your community.

School Service Providers

School is a complex place filled with many different people. There are several different types of people who work with disabled children at the school. This chapter will introduce you to them and what they basically do for your Autistic child.

First, there is the teacher. The teacher leads the classroom instruction and maintains classroom discipline. They have to complete a minimum of four years of college before they can teach in a classroom.

Second, there is the paraprofessional or teacher's aide. They either have completed either two years of college or are currently attending college in some cases. They can be assigned to the classroom in general or a particular student on a full-time basis.

Third, Special Education teacher is a teacher trained to work with disabled kids. They often have certification in a particular field of Special Education. They have each child for varying amounts of time during the day and school subjects. They could have a bachelor's or master's degree.

Fourth, the individual school or the school district has therapists. Depending on the I.E.P., it determines how much time they spend with the child. They could specialize in speech therapy, occupational (small motor skills) therapy, and physical therapy.

Fifth, the school nurse dispenses medication and treats sick and injured children. They are assigned to the individual school or sometimes in rare circumstances a particular disabled child.

Sixth, the school psychologist counsels or evaluates individual students for Special Education services. They help children with their problems.

Finally, each school has a social worker assigned to it in most cases. They work with both the parent and student to help the child reach their full potential both full academic and personal potential. Their supportive role takes many diverse forms and can vary from situation to situation.

Your child's school is part of your team to help you educate your child. Each team player has an important role in educating and preparing your disabled child until adulthood.

Educational Needs

Once your child is diagnosed with Asperger Syndrome, your child is entitled to a free public education until age 21 years old. It falls under federal and state laws. The educational service is dependent upon your local school and school district.

Once your child is diagnosed, you need to inform your child's school or school district dependent upon your child's age. This action needs to be done in writing. I recommend sending it via postal system. There are several key pieces of information that you should write in the letter.

1. First, you need to include your child's name, age, and current grade level (if applicable).
2. Your child's current assigned school and teacher (if applicable).
3. Your child's diagnosis and the doctor who diagnosed your child. This is so your child can receive appropriate testing and placement.
4. Any current problems your child is facing academic wise while attending the school. This action is to give the school an idea of what is happening.

5. You need to have it in writing that you are requesting an evaluation for Special Education services.

Once they receive your letter, they face time limits to complete certain tasks. This includes the school's evaluation, written I.E.P. and I.E.P. conference itself.

The school has to evaluate both your child's functioning and academic levels. I know you have a diagnosis from the doctor. However, they examined your child for a particular diagnosis. Your child's school will evaluate your child for how their disability impacts their education and learning process.

An I.E.P. is a common abbreviation for Individual Education Plan. It is the written document provided by the school outlining your child's educational and therapeutic services for a given amount of time per day, week, and school year.

Your child's educational service refers to the classroom placement(s) and any adaptations that they receive. Educational services can happen in one or more classrooms throughout the school day. The placement is dependent on your Autistic child's needs and capabilities.

The classroom placement is based on the least restrictive environment principle. It is based on the classroom which fits your child's needs with the least adaptations. There is no one size fits all approach to any placement for a disability.

The least restrictive setting according to law is the mainstream or inclusion classroom. Your child will be educated with normal developing children. Your child will be given adaptations which will allow them to participate in classroom activities. Your Autistic child may or may not have a paraprofessional assigned to them. It depends on your child and their academic and behavioral challenges.

The most restricted classroom setting is the self contained classroom. All the children assigned to the classroom are disabled and have an I.E.P. It is when a disabled child receives instruction in one small special education classroom. There is a teacher and one or more assigned paraprofessionals to the classroom.

The resource room combines both the mainstream classroom placement and Special Education. A student comes for a specific class or subject matter for a certain amount of time per day or week. Subjects can include reading, mathematics, language arts, and study skills. Students can sometimes take tests there, too.

The two most restricted settings are hospitalization and homebound instruction. Usually, the disabled child is pretty ill or disabled and unable to attend school. A child will receive a small number of hours per week on homebound instruction. Hospitalization combines both an intensive academic and therapeutic method which can be day or in stay hospital care.

Worked into your child's school day are any therapy sessions given by a trained professional. The services can include physical therapy, speech therapy, and occupational therapy.

Legally, your Autistic child can attend school for free until age 21 years old. Your child can be prepared for the workforce through a job coach while also still getting a high school education.

Your Asperger Syndrome child is entitled to a free and appropriate education up until age 21. It first starts out as early intervention services and preschool. Then, it leads to your child entering kindergarten. The I.E.P. your child receives along the way is dependent upon their own abilities.

Your Asperger Syndrome child's classroom placement might vary from school year to school year depending on their academic needs. A particular type of classroom placement might work one year, but it could create problems during the next school year.

You will find a variety of different classroom placement combinations within Special Education and Autistic kids. One approach might work for one disabled child and would not work for another disabled child even with the same diagnosis. The ideal classroom placement under FAPE takes into consideration your child and how they learn.

You can disagree with a particular placement if you believe it is not in your child's best interests. It should not be done in a confrontational manner. It should be done in a dialogue situation in which both of you discuss your feelings about the classroom placement being considered. You should be well prepared if you try to contest a particular placement on your research and knowledge of your child.

There are things you can suggest or things that can make it better for your child at school. Some of your ideas may work in a classroom and some may not work at all.

You may hear about a shadow or one on one aide for an Autistic child from another parent. It could happen. However, the school district has strict guidelines before issuing a shadow aid for a disabled child. To request one, you need to do your homework and research regarding your child.

Is inclusion for your child? It really should depend upon their academic needs. It should also not be entirely based on your disabled child needing more socialization with non disabled students. If your child struggles in a particular academic area, it is probably better your child goes to at least the resource room for extra help.

The school assigns more than one disabled student typically to a classroom. Some will have an I.E.P. and some will have a Section 504 document. In addition, there can be more than one disability classification in the classroom.

Inclusion works when the mainstream teacher has the proper classroom supports and training in place. It takes more than just an I.E.P. to make a make a classroom placement work. It takes someone willing and able to implement it.

A good inclusion teacher is a team player. They are willing to incorporate a disabled child's I.E.P. into their lesson plans for an individual student. They do not have to do it for their entire classroom. However, they find a way to modify the classroom material towards a particular student's learning needs.

Also, they know when they need help in a particular area. They know both their strengths and weaknesses in different curriculum areas. If they need help, they are willing to approach someone else for help and guidance.

An identified disabled child is entitled to a free and appropriate education until age 21 years old. The academic and therapeutic services are dependent on your child and their capabilities.

There are even job coaches for disabled teens decide that they want to work and are capable of working. They will teach your disabled teen the skills needed to get and keep a job. This is done through the school district or an outside agency for free or a very minimal fee depending on the area.

When your disabled child becomes a high school student, they enter a program to prepare for adulthood. The program is called a transition plan. A transition plan is when the school maps out the steps to prepare your child for adulthood.

College Advice

As with most high school kids, Asperger Syndrome kids do dream of going to college. They could also select a career field which requires a high school degree to work in it. College can create some really interesting challenges for your kid. There is help there for your Asperger Syndrome teen.

At the college or university level, the Individual Education Plan does not exist. However, it does not mean that your teen will not receive help at college. Your disabled teen will qualify for a Section 504 document. It will help them receive help with their college classes. The services come through the disabled services office on campus.

When you start your college searches with your sophomore and junior students, you need to take much more into consideration. You have to think about is the campus the right fit for your Asperger Syndrome teen's needs.

Pay attention to the college dormitory policies. Some colleges and universities can be quite restrictive regarding the usage of them by the students. Some might have the dorms restricted to certain college years because of the lack of available dormitory space.

Does the college offer themed dormitory floors? This can help your Asperger Syndrome teen fit in better with his or her college peers. The reason is that they will have something in common with your disabled teen.

You should closely examine the class size of common classes on campus. Some colleges might make some lecture classes have a larger number of students. As a result, those classes could be in an auditorium like setting.

How are the classes structured for your teen's major? How many courses are lecture? How many are hands on learning experiences? You should find the college with the right mix of courses to match your Asperger Syndrome teen's learning style. By matching a college to your disabled teen's learning style, you could improve their chance of having a successful college career.

What clubs and activities are available on campus? Are there any clubs matching your teen's interests? These can help your teen socialize and meet new friends as a college student.

If you are in doubt about your teen's ability to handle college, you should register them for your local community college first. Your teen might have the academic ability to handle college, but they might not have the maturity or ability to handle life on a college campus.

Before your college student starts school, work on their independence skills. There will be things which will not come automatically to your Asperger Syndrome teen. You need to teach them how to do laundry, budget money, reading bus schedules and budget their time wisely. Teaching them this skill will help you worry less while they are attending college.

After your teen selects the college to attend, contact the Disabled Services office on campus. Find out what documentation is needed to get your teen services through them. This should be done well before the academic year starts, so the Section 504 paperwork is in place to help your teen.

The college years can be a tricky time for Asperger Syndrome teens and young adults. With the right preparations and thoughts, there is a good chance your teen can handle college.

Marriage Advice

Disabilities can be difficult on a marriage. It can make common marriage problems worse at times. How can you make your marriage work?

I discovered the most important thing is communication between you. You need to set time aside each day to talk about important matters on your marriage and personal life. It could include current events or news issues. It helps each of you feel like an adult at least one point during the day.

It is also important to discuss issues regarding your child or children. It could be school, home, or community matters. You could notice a problem with your child and need ideas for solutions. Your spouse might have some ideas how to help your child or an issue. Besides, it could save a future argument by discussing an issue early.

Second, set aside one night each week for date night if possible. It could happen at home or in the community. It helps remind you of what you enjoy most about being with your spouse or significant other. It is enjoying being together. Talk about anything other than the kids during date night.

By taking setting time aside as a couple, it can help reduce the stress on the marriage. It is pretty stressful at times raising a disabled child.

However, it is always an idea to make the marriage a priority at least one time during the week.

Third, you need to coordinate schedules. It helps in planning how therapies and activities in making transportation work. If one partner feels like they have all the work, this attitude can create tension and problems.

Fourth, do not forget your non disabled children. It is easy for them to get lost in the middle of planning for a disabled child with the therapies involved in helping your child. Set aside time each week for some time for normal developing child without your disabled child being present.

Fifth, you have to always remember that it is stressful for the both of you raising a disabled child. It can be both rewarding and pretty frustrating at times depending on the situation at hand. If they are becoming frustrated easy, ask them to take a walk outside just to calm down. Let them know it is not a punishment, but it is to give them a needed break.

Sixth, never criticize your spouse in front of your children or even just your disabled child. You should do it in private in another room with the door closed. If there is a difference in opinions, discuss the matter out and ask about their feelings on the matter. By following this simple advice, it can do wonders for your marriage.

Seventh, take advantage of respite care when you qualify for it. It can give you a much needed break every now and then. It can also do wonders for your marriage at times. This service is offered through an agency. It can be a family member or an outside person. They get paid through the agency to provide the service to you.

Eighth, your spouse could have some denial issues. Your spouse may have Asperger Syndrome himself or herself. Asperger Syndrome was not recognized in the United States until the 1990s by the medical community. As a result, he or she might view your Asperger Syndrome child or teen as just being a normal child or teen.

Finally, share household chores. Ask your spouse to help you around the house. Let them know you would appreciate the help. Tell them it would help you have more energy for them in a day.

If you are remarrying after divorce or death of a spouse, you need to make sure they are fine with raising a disabled child. Not all individuals or step parents can handle the responsibilities of raising one. They should know you have a disabled child and be able to ask questions before making on a final decision to marry you or not. It can save you from having a divorce situation.

You have to be patient at times with your new spouse in the beginning. Everyone makes mistakes in the beginning or misunderstands a situation with your disabled child.

Raising a disabled child is not easy. By following some simple rules, you can ease the strain on your marriage and have less tension between you and your spouse. By following these ideas, you could possibly save yourself from a divorce situation. However, there are cases out there is no method from preventing a divorce from happening.

Raising Siblings

Having a brother or sister is not always easy for a child. Life gets even more complicated and difficult for a child when they have a disabled sibling. What are some things that you can do as a parent to make life easier for your normal development child?

First, set time aside for your non disabled child each day or week. It is easy to be busy with your disabled child's activities because of their many different needs. The time and the activity are up to you and your child. You could plan the activity in advance or you could plan on the day in particular.

Second, create an activity schedule calendar for each child, and you should create a master schedule for everyone in the family. Outline the important events during each day because it shows that he or she is important person and does not feel like an outsider.

Third, you should not consider your normal child a free babysitter for your disabled child when they become a teenager. They might enjoy spending time with each other. However, they might resent having always to be responsible for their sibling as a teen. Just as any babysitter would get paid, your teen deserves to be paid to babysit also.

Fourth, let your kids develop their own sibling relationship among themselves. Unless it is an unhealthy one, let them develop it. It will make your life easier in not having to be a referee among them. Your interference could create more problems than you think.

Fifth, remember to praise your child when things are great with both kids. Kids love positive feedback when they attempt to try something new. Praise is a very encouraging factor in their development as a child. Giving them praise also gives them a positive sense of self.

Sixth, encourage them not to tease or mock your child. Also, encourage them not to be around kids who tease, bully, or mock disabled children. It is easy to ignore children who are different. However, it can create uneasy or hurt feelings in themselves and the entire family.

Seventh, let your normal developing child sign up for activities. This will help them have a normal childhood. If your child requires a lot of outside therapy, find ways to get them to the scout meetings, dance classes, or sports practices. This will also help them not have any guilt feelings about their disabled sibling.

Eighth, find activities that they could participate in together at their own functioning levels. Some siblings will love to find ways to enjoy doing things together whether in a community setting, sport, or some form club activity.

Ninth, there can at times be some sibling rivalry between your Asperger Syndrome child and your normal developing child. Your normal developing child could use your disabled child's disability to attack them. You have to remind your normal child to remind them that it is not nice to pick on someone's weaknesses because it could happen to them one day at school.

Finally, remember your normal developing child has their good days and bad days. You have to have a minimal amount of patience with them on their bad days. You also need to appreciate their good days, too.

Being a parent of a disabled child is a tough job. However, it is an even more difficult job being the sibling of a disabled child. With the right parenting approach, your normal developing child will turn out great and have a wonderful relationship with their disabled sibling.

Support Groups

Your child was just diagnosed with Autism. You begin to wonder about how to help them with their daily life. You think about their future. When you think about these things, it tends to get very overwhelming for you.

I discovered long ago the power of having a support group in your life. It could include your friends and family. It can also include strangers with children diagnosed with Autism.

The thing is that support groups take many different forms. It can be geared towards all age group of parents or just a specific group. It depends on the individuals involved with it.

In some areas, you might find a several support groups for different disabilities. On the other hand, you might only find one large support group for parents of all disabled kids. It just depends on the region of the country in which you live.

For parents, a support group can be really beneficial to you. It can help you with some of the common problems your child will face in life. It can even give you ideas on how to parent better your disabled child at times. The amount of things that you learn at the meeting depends on the topic.

Support groups can be great for your Autistic child's siblings. Often, these groups can be located through your child's school or disability organization. In these support groups, they will find peers who know what they are going through in life. They can also learn how to cope with their sibling's disability characteristics better.

One of the best things in life happens to be support groups for a parent of a disabled child. You can learn many different things from them. You can also find the support that you need on a regular basis. In there, you will discover people from a variety of different backgrounds, but you will find one common experience through the love of a disabled child.

About Your Child's Future

I know you worry about your child's future as an Asperger Syndrome individual. It is a common worry among any parent with any child disabled or not disabled. As the years progress, you wonder what your child's life will be like once they reach adulthood. Honestly, knowing about your child's future is the most difficult question to answer.

I learned that there are so many different life factors in determining what their future holds for them. From my own experience, no two disabled children turn out the same given the same set of opportunities out there.

The best advice that I could give you is take advantage of the free education given to your child. You will find some of the best trained people in dealing with your child's disability work in the public school system. However, it may seem hard to believe at times during your child's education.

Your child's future depends a lot on you and your spouse. Everything you teach them influences the person who they become in life. It also influences how they perceive themselves. I know there are times that you want to give up on things. It can be very frustrating at times dealing with a disabled child. However, it is the most rewarding job of them all to see them develop slowly into an adult.

Read to your child on a regular basis just like you would any child. Choose an interesting book with an interesting plot or learning activity. You can find these books in your local public library. By exposing your child to books, you give them an opportunity to learn something new.

Each person views the world in a different way than another person. The same holds true with the disabled population. Each one can be a true gift to the world if prepared and taught right.

Your child will learn from their teachers, classmates, friends, and age peers. Each interaction will teach them about people. The information will be sometimes good and sometimes bad. It depends on how you teach them to interact with other people and social situations.

There are so many different job opportunities out there for the disabled. It depends on your child and their capabilities on which career path that they will take in life. Once they are in the right career, you will find that they have a great enthusiasm for the field. Their bosses and job coach will help them be the best employee that they can be in their job.

The best thing you could do for yourself and your spouse is find the best support network you can. It does not have to be financial. It is just for moral support. It can work wonders at times when you need it the most in life.

Live each day as if it is an adventure. You never know in which direction your child's disability will lead the two of you. They will have good days. They will have bad days. Just take each day as a new learning experience in your child's life. School does not end after you graduate from school. School graduation marks the beginning of a new style of learning in your life.

Life is never easy. I will be the first to admit it. However, you have the unique opportunity to shape the life of a disabled person. Not everyone has the opportunity to do so in life. Always remember that your disabled child is a special gift to you and the world. In many ways, you will find your disabled child a blessing in your life.

Afterword

I started Practical Asperger Syndrome Handbook after spending much time around parents of disabled children for the past almost fourteen years. I noticed many of the same questions and concerns that they had for their Asperger Syndrome child.

It came after being a volunteer parent educator for the past almost 14 years. I have worked with probably over a thousand different families with disabled children.

In addition, some of my friends have Asperger Syndrome. They are disabled because of an extra chromosome, but they have the biggest hearts of them all when it comes to love. They are also very hard working and care about doing the best job that they can in whatever they do in life.

My biggest joy is the knowledge that a disabled child will be prepared for adulthood to their level of ability. Each child has a gift for perceiving the world differently than another person might in the same situation.

I know it is confusing right now on what to do to help your child. Follow your instincts and your heart. Your heart will help you in raising your Asperger Syndrome child to adulthood.

I know you will find the book useful in your quest to help your Asperger Syndrome child. I know I covered many basic things about it. However, I meant this book as an introduction into the wonderful world of Asperger Syndrome children.

Glossary

ABA: Also known as Applied Behavioral Analysis. An intensive time therapeutic method used to educate young Autistic kids. It is expensive.

Applied Behavioral Analysis: See ABA.

Behavior Modification Plan: A written plan developed to help a teacher work on a disabled child's problem behavior areas.

Charter School: An independent publically funded school providing an alternative to public school education. The school does not charge tuition to the parents. Some offer a themed curriculum.

Developmental Pediatrician: A doctor who works with children with behavioral and learning issues from infancy to early adulthood.

Early Intervention: Therapy services given to developmentally disabled children under the age of three years old.

Homebound Instruction: It happens when a disabled is so severe that they are unable to attend school. The amount of instruction provided by a teacher is limited to a small amount of hours per week.

Inclusion: Refers to the disabled child being placed in a regular classroom with non disabled peers. This is the least restrictive environment placement.

Job Coach: A person who trains a disabled person for a job. Typically breaks down a large job task into smaller parts.

Least Restrictive Environment: Also known as LRE. It refers to the classroom placement which fits the needs of your child. It can range from homebound instruction to an inclusion classroom situation.

Magnet School: A themed curriculum school offered by a school district or county. Has sometimes a selective enrollment criteria and limited admissions process to it.

Mainstream: Another name for an inclusion classroom placement at school.

Paraprofessional: Often called a teacher's aide. Can either be assigned to an entire classroom or a single student for all or part of the school day?

Resource room: A disabled child will come to this classroom for certain subjects or a certain amount of time per day or week. Typically, it is for reading, mathematics, and writing. It can include study skills.

Respite Care: A trained paid individual comes to your home for a certain amount of hours to give you a break.

Section 504: A document which allows a disabled child to have the modifications they need to attend school. It comes from an unfunded federal government mandate. It is for a disabled student who does not qualify for Special Education or an I.E.P. under federal and state government regulations.

Service Animal: Often is a trained dog who works with disabled individuals to help with certain daily tasks.

Shadow Aide: One on one paraprofessional assigned to a disabled student.

Social Skills Training: A group speech therapy session in which an Autistic student learns how to hold a basic conversation.

Special Education: An educational program for identified disabled students at school. A student is evaluated to see if they qualify. Each student is given an I.E.P.

Specials: Refers to art, music, gym class. Some disabled students are only mainstreamed for these classes during their school day.

Transition Plan: A plan to prepare a teenager for the adult world after high school graduation. It includes work place goals after high school.

Wrap Around Services: Therapy and counseling given to a disabled student outside school. It is meant to complement and enhance school services given to your child.

Resources

I have included a list of websites that I have found useful over the years. I refer people all the time to them. I have no professional association with their organization, company, or website.

ABA: www.abainternational.org

About Autism: autism.about.com

About Pediatrics: pediatrics.about.com

Asperger Syndrome: www.aspergersyndrome.org

Autism Education: www.difflearn.com

Autism Society: www.autism-society.org

Cafemom: www.cafemom.com

CDC: www.cdc.gov

CHADD: www.chadd.org

Charter Schools: www.uscharterschools.org

Disability.gov: www.disability.gov

Easter Seals: www.easterseals.org

Family Voices: www.familyvoices.org

Food Allergy Initiative: www.faiusa.org

Generation Rescue: www.generationrescue.org

Learning Disability: www.ldonline.org

LOVAAS Therapy Method: www.lovaas.com

NARHA Inc.: www.narha.org

National Agricultural: Library: www.nutrition.gov

NICHCY Education Center: www.nichcy.org

Social Security Administration: www.ssa.gov

Special Education: www.seriweb.com

Special Olympics: www.specialolympics.org

Talk Autism: www.talkautism.com

Teach2Talk: www.teach2talk.com

TheARC: www.thearc.org

Very Special Arts: www.vsarts.org

WebMD: www.webmd.com

Wrightslaw: www.wrightslaw.com

About the Author

Dawn Lucan is a disabled freelance writer who lives on the East Coast. She is the founder and creator of the Memory series which is a series of social stories books for preschoolers through high school graduation. She enjoys reading and watching movies when she is not writing. Her author website can be located at www.toyboxunlimited.com.